I0115214

Erectile Dysfunction Protocol Book

Copyright 2015

by Dan Purser MD

http://www.drpursertestosteroneoptions.com

My Legal Protection

This book is for education and entertainment purposes only! Please do not use the information contained in this book to treat yourself. Please consult with a knowledgeable physician in your area before starting any treatment as might possibly be suggested in this book. I will not be held responsible if something goes wrong. So BE CAREFUL!

Thank you.

Dan Purser MD

Foreword

I see so many men who have ED (erectile dysfunction) and have been given the usual drug for it – the little blue pill (sildenafil). Boom.

That's it. No work-up. Minimal evaluation. These men were asked just a few questions during their visit. I don't get it.

The FDA (in the Physician's Desk Reference™) and the AAFP (American Academy of Family Practice) and ACIM (American College of Internal Medicine) all advise in their journals to at least to do an evaluation, physical examination and check a testosterone level. As far as I can see these usually are not done.

So the guy gets the "little blue pill" and gets shown the door (after he pays of course), but the underlying problems were never addressed.

That's what I do – dive deeper – get to root causes.

But I can't get into this too much here – but am going to discuss those options along with some more natural options to assist in your ED problems.

Thank you so much for purchasing this book!

Want to Connect With Dr. Purser?

For men's information on testosterone issues and their medical problems and a more thoughtful approach to men's problems and to download some awesome REPORTS:

http://www.drpursergift.com

The REPORTS You Get!

YOU NEED THESE -- PLUS YOUR BONUS LAB REPORT!

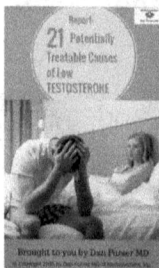

Low levels of testosterone can be treated naturally & optimally in the right situations.	Questions I hear all the time from men regarding their low libido & testosterone. YOU SHOULD ASK THESE!	An AMAZING LIST every man should own -- all REFERENCED! NO FOOLING.	Detailed Info on Lab Levels & Where to Get them CHEAP when your doc won't!

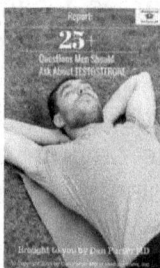

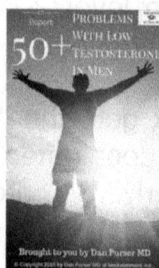

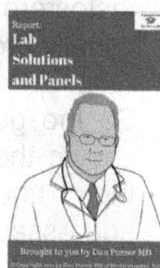

© Copyright by Dan Purser MD of
Medutainment, Inc.

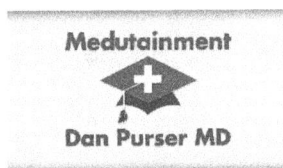

Chapters

Chapter One

What the Experts Are Saying

"Testosterone first?

Before Viagra appeared on the scene in 1998 and transformed the treatment of erectile dysfunction, testosterone was an important medical therapy for it. Testosterone is central in the male sexual response, including the desire for sex and the mechanics of triggering an erection.

To be sure, getting more of this hormone isn't a universal solution for ED. Some men with erectile problems have perfectly normal amounts of testosterone. Many doctors won't consider prescribing testosterone unless certain other symptoms are also present, such as decreased desire for sex (libido) and fatigue. And boosting testosterone doesn't always improve erections. But it is an option on the table for men with low testosterone.

"It's well established that testosterone by itself, for men with sexual dysfunction that includes erectile dysfunction, can improve erections in the majority of men who take it," says Dr. Abraham Morgentaler, an associate clinical professor of urology at Harvard-affiliated Beth Israel Deaconess Medical Center.

Dr. Morgentaler is also the founder and director of Men's Health Boston, which treats many men with low testosterone. At the clinic, "our first choice for men who have low testosterone and erection problems is to give them testosterone and not sildenafil," says Dr. Morgentaler, the author of Testosterone for Life. "Improved doesn't always mean adequate, though, so, it is not unusual to add sildenafil or a similar medication if a man still is not satisfied with the quality of his erection with testosterone therapy alone."

One potential advantage to the "testosterone first" approach is that it could make it unnecessary to take a pill in the anticipation of a sexual encounter. Also, men with low testosterone and symptoms may experience extra benefits of testosterone replacement, such as more "pep" and more desire for sex in the first place."[1]

And this is just one (though admittedly highly respected) group of experts.

It's a widespread issue.

The Problem

So you're a man who's not doing very well in bed and you tell your doctor you have sexual problems?

What usually happens next?

Knee jerk reaction is most doctors will offer you Viagra™ or Cialis™. (Notice that I did not say doctors check your testosterone or LH or FSH levels, but that the first thing they do is to start you on Viagra™.)

Why?

Because this approach is quick and easy and gets you out of their crowded overbooked office.

It's also incorrect and is very ignorant (again IMHO). They should at the least check your free and total testosterone and LH/FSH levels. I believe this occurs because most doctors have NO idea what's an appropriate level of testosterone for a man.

What is ED?

ED (Erectile Dysfunction) is caused by many different things -- a multitude -- but there are a few basic root causes that need to be properly dealt with before improvement can occur.

What ED is NOT: Lack of Viagra®/Cialis®/Levitra®

What ED Is...

What we're mostly talking about here is "mild ED" – which includes the feeling that "you're not as hard as you could be" and often responds to natural remedies.

Chapter Two

Causes of ED

Male sexual arousal is a complex process that involves the brain, hormones, emotions, nerves, muscles and blood vessels. Erectile dysfunction can result from a problem with any of these.

Likewise, stress and mental health concerns can cause or worsen erectile dysfunction.

Sometimes a combination of physical and psychological issues causes erectile dysfunction. For instance, a minor physical condition that slows your sexual response might cause anxiety about maintaining an erection. The resulting anxiety can lead to or worsen erectile dysfunction.

Physical causes of erectile dysfunction

In most cases, erectile dysfunction is caused by something physical. Common causes include:

- Trauma
- Heart disease
- Clogged blood vessels (atherosclerosis)
- High cholesterol
- High blood pressure
- Diabetes
- Obesity
- Metabolic syndrome — a condition

involving increased blood pressure, high insulin levels, body fat around the waist and high cholesterol
- Parkinson's disease
- Multiple sclerosis
- ALS (Amyotrophic Lateral Sclerosis)
- Peyronie's disease — development of scar tissue inside the penis
- Hypogonadism
- Anterior Pituitary Dysfunction
- Certain prescription medications
- Tobacco use
- Alcoholism and other forms of substance abuse
- Sleep disorders
- Treatments for prostate cancer or enlarged prostate
- Surgeries or injuries that affect the pelvic area or spinal cord

Psychological causes of erectile dysfunction

The brain plays a key role in triggering the series of physical events that cause an erection, starting with feelings of sexual excitement. A number of things can interfere with sexual feelings and cause or worsen erectile dysfunction. These include:

- Depression, anxiety or other mental health conditions
- Stress
- Relationship problems due to stress, poor communication or other concerns[2]

Chapter Three

Treatment Options

Why You Need to See Your Doctor[3]

It's critical to be evaluated by your doctor because ED may be a sign of additional health problems. For example, if you have heart disease, you can take a number of steps that will likely improve both your heart health and your ED. This includes lowering your cholesterol, reducing your weight, or taking medications to unclog your blood vessels.

Standard treatments for ED include lifestyle changes, such as:

- Exercising
- Losing weight
- Stopping smoking
- Curbing alcohol intake

Non-drug treatments for ED

- Penile vacuum pumps
- Penile implants
- Blood vessel surgery

First You Should Optimize Your Testosterone Levels

Most of the respected medical experts in this area of practice (I believe) think you should "normalize" [I say optimize] your tes levels (serum Total Testosterone of 800-1200 ng/dl) in the best and most appropriate way for you first (if you want to have more kids do this via HCG injections, or if not – via a quality compounded tes cream or testosterone cypionate injection).

NATURAL SOLUTIONS

Natural Solution #1: Panax Ginseng[4]

Called the "herbal Viagra," Panax ginseng ("Korean red ginseng") has solid research behind it[5]. Researchers reviewed seven studies of red ginseng and ED in 2008[6]. Dosages ranged from 600 to 1,000 mg three times daily. They concluded there was "suggestive evidence for the effectiveness of red ginseng in the treatment of erectile dysfunction."

Amazon® carries a NOW™ brand of Panax Ginseng that is available for this purpose.

Natural Solution #2: Rhodiola Rosea[7]

One small study also indicated Rhodiola rosea may be helpful[8]. Twenty-six out of 35 men were given 150 to 200 mg a day for three months. They experienced substantially improved sexual function.

Amazon® also carries a NOW™ brand of Rhodiola rosea that is available for this purpose.

Natural Solution #3: DHEA[9]

Dehydroepiandrosterone (DHEA) is a natural hormone produced by the adrenal glands and testicles. It can be converted to both estrogen and testosterone in the body. Scientists make the dietary supplement from wild yam or soy.

The influential Massachusetts Male Aging Study[10] showed that men with ED were more likely to have low levels of DHEA. Forty men with ED participated in another study published in 1999, in which half received 50 mg DHEA and half received a placebo once a day for six months. Those receiving the DHEA were more likely to achieve and maintain an erection.

You have to be very careful on DHEA manufacturing as many brands are extremely weak and when patients take it their levels do not change (making you wonder what's in there). Also when your blood level is high enough you'll possibly develop a facial cystic acne lesion (usually starts out as just one) –

this means it's time to cut back to one or two a week. But Amazon® carries a Life Extension™ brand of DHEA at 50 mg a capsule that is available and can be trusted for this purpose.

Natural Solution #4: L-ARGININE[11]

L-arginine is an amino acid naturally present in the body. It helps make nitric oxide. Nitric oxide relaxes blood vessels to facilitate a successful erection. Researchers studied the effects of L-arginine on ED in 1999[12]. Thirty-one percent of men with ED taking 5 grams of L-arginine a day experienced significant improvements in sexual function.

A second study showed that L-arginine combined with pycnogenol, a plant product from tree bark, restored sexual ability to 80 percent of participants after two months. Ninety-two percent had restored sexual ability after three months[13]. Another study in Japan, using Prelox® (combination of pycnogenol and L-arginine) showed supplementation enhanced sperm volume and concentration, motility, vitality and morphology significantly versus placebo. The Fertility Index rose to normal values during treatment. e-NOS activity in sperm was also elevated. No adverse effects were reported[14].

The other MAIN function of L-arginine is in the production of testosterone – you must have it to make testosterone. Period.

Definitely something you MUST add if you

have ED.

I love the L-Arginine efficacy and vitamin blend in the Synergy™ product Pro-Argi-9® (I am not a distributor nor do I profit off the sale of this product – I just like the quality and use it myself). But if obtaining that product is too complicated you can also get a very high quality 1,000 mg (1 gram) version of L-arginine here through our affiliate link.

Natural Solution #5: ACUPUNCTURE

Though studies are mixed, many show positive results when acupuncture is used to treat ED. A 1999 study[15], for example, found that acupuncture improved the quality of erections and restored sexual activity in 39 percent of participants.

A later study published in 2003 reported that 21 percent of ED patients who received acupuncture had improved erections[16]. Other studies have shown conflicting results, but this treatment has potential and may work for you.

Amazon™ offers a home acupuncture kit for ED that should give you fun and success.

Natural Solution #6: ZINC

Several studies have shown that zinc supplements (especially for men who are low in zinc or who have kidney disease), can work wonders and help with both testosterone and thyroid function and production, and erectile dysfunction[17].

You can purchase a helpful <u>50 mg gluconated version here</u> through our Amazon affiliate link (seriously).

Natural Solution #7: POMEGRANATE JUICE

Drinking antioxidant-rich pomegranate juice has been shown to have numerous health benefits, including a reduced risk for heart disease and high blood pressure. Does pomegranate juice also protect against ED? No proof exists, but results of a study published in 2007 were promising. The authors of this small-scale pilot study called for additional research, saying that larger-scale studies might prove <u>pomegranate juice</u>'s effectiveness against erectile dysfunction[18]. "I tell my patients to drink it," says Espinosa. "It could help ED, and even if it doesn't, it has other health benefits."

Natural Solution #8: YOHIMBE

Before Viagra and the other prescription erectile dysfunction drugs became available, doctors sometimes prescribed a derivative of the herb yohimbe (yohimbine hydrochloride) to their patients suffering from ED. But experts say the medication is not particularly effective, and it can cause jitteriness and other problems. "It's not a great drug," says McCullough. "And I suspect the herb is not as potent as the pharmaceutical version." What's more, evidence shows that yohimbe is associated with high blood pressure, anxiety, headache, and other health problems. Experts discourage its use. (I wouldn't advise this one as I think it's not medically safe to use.)

Natural Solution #9: HORNY GOAT WEED

Horny goat weed and related herbs have purportedly been treatments for sexual dysfunction for years. Italian researchers found that the main compound in horny goat weed, called icariin, acted in a similar way as drugs like Viagra. There was an even more advantageous study performed at the University or California, San Francisco Medical Center that showed great activity of icariin[19].

Source Naturals™, an excellent brand, has a horny goat weed capsule that is reported to be excellent and has great reviews.

Natural Solution #10: GINKGO BILOBA

Known primarily as a treatment for cognitive decline, ginkgo has also been used to treat erectile dysfunction -- especially cases caused by the use of certain antidepressant medications. But the evidence isn't very convincing. One 1998 study published in the Journal of Sex and Marital Therapy found that it did work[20]. But a more rigorous study, published in Human Pharmacology in 2002, failed to replicate this finding. "Ginkgo has come out of fashion in the past few years," says Ronald Tamler, MD, assistant professor of medicine and co-director of the men's health program at Mount Sinai Medical Center in New York City. "That's because it doesn't do much. I can say that in my practice, I have not seen ginkgo work -- ever."

After that ever so glowing last statement by Dr. Tamler if you'd still like to try some – this is a good variety by Life Extension® available on Amazon®.

Natural Solution #11: Fish Oil

ED usually is a cardiovascular issue – my thought has always been that fish oil (DHA and EPA) is used to prevent sudden cardiac death. Uhhh, and when you're having lots of fun sex ('cause your ED has pretty much resolved) you may be having some pretty fun "activities" and it would not be cool to die from a sudden cardiac event[21].

You need to take an average of 2,500 mg per day of good high quality fish oil to gain this protection. I usually use **Source Naturals™ ArcticPure® Omega-3 1125 Fish Oil** -- it contains 1,125 mg per capsule of EPA + DHA requiring you to just take two a day. And rest assured it's safe -- it is both pharmaceutical grade and molecularly distilled (my two major requirements with fish oil).

Natural Solution #12: CRESTOR® OR SIMVASTATIN

Statins? Really? These are not natural, right? Yes, they are not natural.

BUT hear me out.

These two statins have been shown in several clinical trials to cause plaque regression.

What?

Plaque regression. This is where plaque in the arteries (such as in your heart or brain or penis), melts away.

So if you have angina, coronary artery disease, or plaque issues you should be on a statin – and these two (Crestor®[22] and simvastatin[23]) – are the only ones to my knowledge that work in performing this function.

Now sildenafil works still in this situation (sometimes) but, for the most part, only in men who have circulatory problems – i.e. men with plaque in their penis.

So it only makes sense to try one of these two statins.

My rules on these statins?

1. Take with CoQ10 to prevent the myalgias (I prefer Qunol®—2 a day).

2. Your doctor needs to monitor you closely (liver, muscles and kidneys).

3. Start low and go slow but you need to eventually get to maximum dose for this to work.

Natural Solution #13: βHCG (Human Chorionic Gonadotropin)

βHCG is produced in both the placenta of pregnant women (where it further advances the sexual development of the unborn child) and the pituitary stalks of both men and women. Let me please be clear about this because you men for some reason assume that βHCG is a female hormone only. IT IS NOT. It is a male hormone too (so any nipple tenderness is not from the βHCG but from the aromatization of testosterone to estradiol).

βHCG is actually just a bunch of LH (luteinizing hormone) and FSH (follicle stimulating hormone), which in turn, are pituitary hormones that stimulate your testicles to make more testosterone and can help with erections.

You should know that βHCG is prescription, tricky to use, is a shot, can be pricey, and your doctor may not be familiar with using or prescribing it.

But know in the PDR® it is FDA approved for "central" (pituitary) hypogonadism use.

Natural Solution #14: CLOMIPHENE CITRATE

Also called Clomid®, it is a SERM.

Wait a what?

A SERM – a Selective Estradiol Reuptake Modulator – meaning it blocks negative estradiol feedback in your hypothalamus thus increasing your LH and FSH which stimulates your testicles[24] to make testosterone and sperm and spermatic fluid and DHEA. It's oral. It's cheap. It IS prescription but it DOES help. It WILL boost your own production.
And it has minimal side effects, too.

All this definitely helps with ED (especially the mild or moderate forms), too.

Natural Solution #15: NO VITAMIN DEFICIENCIES

Vitamin deficiencies are CRITICAL to your health – serious lack of key vitamins can hamper or even inhibit completely your bodies' ability to make testosterone and sperm. And obtain an erection.

In our office we perform intracellular vitamin and micronutrient testing regularly but ask your doctor for this and get it and follow the test's suggestions.

Natural Solution #16: COMPOUNDED TESTOSTERONE CREAM

This is always a Plan B but can definitely help if nothing else works and you have severe enough Primary Hypogonadism. This is DEA controlled and you'll need an evaluation and prescription from your doctor to get.

Natural Solution #17: NIASPAN®

A prescription extended release niacin, Niaspan®, has a film coating that delays release of the niacin, resulting in an absorption over a period of 8–12 hours. The extended release formulations generally reduce vasodilation and flushing side effects, but increase the risk of hepatotoxicity compared to the immediate release forms.

Studies have shown patients need to take up to 2,000 mg a day to get plaque regression (or use with one of the before mentioned two statins[25]), but the plaque regression really does happen. The risk of liver problems and horrible flushing (just about guaranteed) is part of the side effects. You must start with a tiny dose and work up slowly to the 2,000 mg and be closely monitored. The flushing is more like a burning horrible prickly heat that lasts a while (up to 30 minutes) but it also shows that it is working (if you follow a "No Triglyceride/Carb" diet and eat very carefully this won't happen).

And instead of Niaspan® you could just take quick release niacin 250 mg and build up slowly (which could be uncomfortable but is very cheap – I do not advise the "timed-release" or "slow release" versions due to health concerns).

Internet rumors say that taking smaller doses of Niaspan® with sildenafil (Viagra®) will very much enhance the anti-ED benefits of sildenafil. But there have been no studies to justify this claim.

Natural Solution #18: Wife/Girlfriend/Partner

No matter what erectile dysfunction treatment or treatments a man ultimately decides upon, experts say it's important to eat healthfully and to avoid smoking and heavy drinking. In addition, says Lamm, "A loving, receptive, and responsive partner is a home run. After all, this is still a couple's issue."

Natural Solution #19: Proper Diet

No matter what erectile dysfunction treatment or treatments a man ultimately decides upon, the diet is the most important (especially if they lose tummy fat). I do not think, with what we've learned in the last few years, the Atkins Diet is the best option and could be harmful as there's some indication that it may lead to plaque build-up.

See this Google™ search screenshot I took.

Web   Shopping   News   Videos   Images   More ▾   Search tools

About 510,000 results (0.57 seconds)

The prevention and regression of atherosclerotic plaques ...
www.ncbi.nlm.nih.gov/... ▾ National Center for Biotechnology Information ▾
by AA Kalanuria - 2012 - Cited by 9 - Related articles
Sep 25, 2012 - All the risk factors **contribute** to pathogenesis by aggravating the underlying .... The American heart Association provides recommendations for **diet** and lifestyle .... Hibi et al studied effects of statin treatment on **plaque regression** in .... It **does** not appear at the moment that anacetrapib exhibits the side effects ...

Low-carbohydrate Atkins-style diets could increase risk of ...
www.dailymail.co.uk/.../**Low-carb**ohydrate-**Atkins**-style-**diets**-... ▾ Daily Mail ▾
Aug 25, 2009 - Risk: **Low-carb**, high-protein **diets** can cause a build-up of **plaque** in arteries ... Scientists found that **Atkins** style **diets** can **lead** to a 'significant' build up in **plaque** in arteries. .... I may not like it but my liver **does**. .... resulting in a direct and rapid **reduction** in human health which has been well documented by ...

The Dangers of a Low Carb Diet - Peak Testosterone
www.peaktestosterone.com/**Atkins_Low_Carb_Diet**.aspx ▾
Here are a dozen major, research-backed dangers of a **Low Carb Diet**, ... However, there no doubt that the increased cortsiol and other stress hormones that result from **Low Carb Diets** may **contribute** as well. .... where the partipants losetweight and ALL 3 diets showed **plaque regression** simply due .... WHAT LOW T **DOES**:.

[PDF] Regression - espen
www.espen.org/... ▾ European Society for Clinical Nutrition and Metabolism ▾
... Therapy 2010. Current markers for prediction of **plaque regression** ... Med & **Low-carb diets** → more favorable in lipid profile. Low carb. Low carb. Low carb.

Reversal Therapy, a Better Treatment for Heart Disease
www.thedoctorwillseeyounow.com/content/heart/art2027.html ▾
It treats the underlying causes of cholesterol accumulation and **plaque** ... an unhealthy **diet**, lack of exercise, high blood pressure, diabetes and stress. ... which **lead to plaque** rupture and heart attack or narrowing that causes chest pain. ... Make up your mind low fat for cholesterol lowering or **low carb** for weight control?

So I think that Dean Ornish's work on diet (see his newest book, The Spectrum®, as a healthy lifestyle option and good read) and cardiovascular disease and improvement (and plaque regression) as THE BEST DIET option for men with ED.

Chapter Four

Optimize Everything Else

Thyroid – This hormone and level needs to be followed correctly by physicians. In our office and in my training and research we always follow the Free T3 (FT3) level when we adjust thyroid levels. If it's safe cardiovascularly, one should always try to elevate FT3 level to optimal levels (3.8-4.2 ng/dl). Why not? If a patient has to take thyroid, you might as well make sure they take enough, right?

At a FT3 of approximately 4.0, a number of really good things can happen:

1. Plaque regression occurs from arteries (coronary, carotid, and penile, too)[26].
2. You get a big decrease in breast[27] AND lung cancer[28].
3. It's easier to, and you'll have more energy to, exercise and/or have sex or intercourse.
4. Your cholesterol and triglycerides will drop to normal (thus the plaque regression in #1).
5. This can really help with testosterone and sperm production[29] -- sometimes making it normal!

Remember and WARNING – you must take lots of CoQ10 when you take oral thyroid or you will deplete your CoQ10 levels. I see lots of patients who are taking thyroid yet are exhausted all the time. When you start them on a good quality CoQ10 (like Qunol™ – I will have them take 4 or 5 a day the first week, then 2 a day thereafter), 95% of the time they feel dramatically better with more energy and endurance and stamina. Go to Stephen Sinatra MD's website for more information – he's a cardiologist in Boston who is considered by many to be the top expert in the USA on CoQ10 use.

Why the Qunol™? For the myalgias and the myopathy – we believe it's due to the statin using up the CoQ10 in the mitochondria, this then causes the muscles to become inflamed and hurt. I have never seen myalgia or myopathy when the simvastatin is taken with adequate CoQ10.

Aspirin – I'd highly advise half an aspirin every day for anyone who has ED (unless you cannot take due to other medical reasons or your doctor says not to do so).

Vitamins -- get a SpectraCell® to determine what amino acids, vitamins, and minerals you need. It's really critical at this point to make sure you're taking adequate vitamins every day.

Chapter Five

Have Less Frequent Sex

Probably not the answer you want but having less sex can cause you to super charge your love life. At least with ED issues. Not with sperm count issues.

Studies have shown that more frequent sex and orgasm actually increases sperm count and spermatic fluid[30].

All good things.

But less sex let's you build up interest, desire, hormones and erection strength.

Rest does too.

So take it easy and have some fun with your significant other. And relax. Less is sometimes better.

Good luck with your ED!

And if you think this little book has helped, please feel free to leave me a review – it really helps to pay it forward so other men are encouraged to get the help they need.

Bonus Chapter!!

Essential Oils May Also Help Erectile Dysfunction

Below is a list of essential oils that may help impotence symptoms – they would be applied topically at vitaflex points or elsewhere (it varies according to who you talk to -- ask a naturopath or search it online).

The oils listed may stimulate circulation, and may also help to work on underlying emotional issues -- **Clary Sage, Peppermint, Ylang Ylang, Sandalwood, Rose, and Jasmine** may help tackle emotional fears such as depression, performance anxiety, fear of failure, and more. **Ginger Root, Nutmeg, Sandalwood, Black Pepper, and Jasmine** may help to increase blood flow as well as circulation.

You can see more at: www.biosourcenaturals.com/essential-oils-for-impotence (I am not affiliated with these people but really like their work).

Thank you so much for purchasing this book!

Want to Connect With Dr. Purser?

For men's information on testosterone issues and their medical problems and a more thoughtful approach to men's problems and to download some awesome REPORTS:

http://www.drpursergift.com

The REPORTS You Get!

YOU NEED THESE -- PLUS YOUR BONUS LAB REPORT!

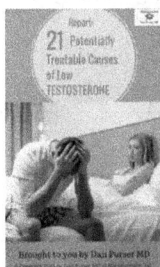

| Low levels of testosterone can be treated naturally & optimally in the right situations. | Questions I hear all the time from men regarding their low libido & testosterone. YOU SHOULD ASK THESE! | An AMAZING LIST every man should own -- all REFERENCED! NO FOOLING. | Detailed Info on Lab Levels & Where to Get them CHEAP when your doc won't! |

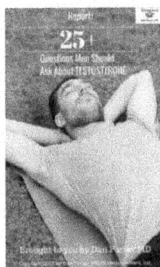

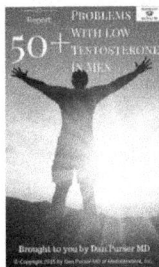

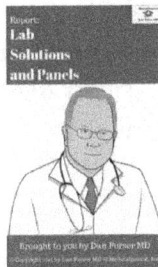

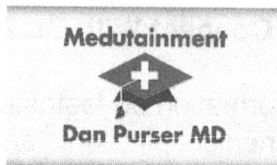

Medutainment

Dan Purser MD

Thank You!

I know you chose to read this book from millions of options, and I really appreciate it. It really does mean a lot to me, and my team that you would read this book that will change your life. If you enjoyed this book, and believe it did help you, <u>please take a moment to leave a review on my Amazon page.</u>

I, Dan Purser MD, personally go over every single review, to make sure my books really are reaching out and helping you. Please help me help you, by leaving a review!

-- Dan Purser MD

References

[1] Accessed 28 April 2015 online at
http://www.health.harvard.edu/blog/a-logical-approach-to-treating-erectile-dysfunction-201211275583
[2] By Mayo Clinic Staff. Causes. Accessed on 20 April 2015 online at http://www.mayoclinic.org/diseases-conditions/erectile-dysfunction/basics/causes/con-20034244
[3] Story, CM. 5 Natural Treatments for Erectile Dysfunction. Accessed 20 April 2015 online at http://www.healthline.com/health/erectile-dysfunction/ed-natural-treatments#Overview1.
[4] Freeman, D. Natural Remedies for Erectile Dysfunction. Accessed 21 April 2015 online at http://www.webmd.com/erectile-dysfunction/features/natural-remedies-for-erectile-dysfunction.
[5] Chan SW. Panax ginseng, Rhodiola rosea and Schisandra chinensis. Int J Food Sci Nutr. 2012 Mar;63 Suppl 1:75-81. doi: 10.3109/09637486.2011.627840.
[6] Jang DJ, Lee MS, et al. Red ginseng for treating erectile dysfunction: a systematic review. Br J Clin Pharmacol. 2008 Oct;66(4):444-50. doi: 10.1111/j.1365-2125.2008.03236.x.
[7] Freeman, D. Natural Remedies for Erectile Dysfunction. Accessed 21 April 2015 online at http://www.webmd.com/erectile-dysfunction/features/natural-remedies-for-erectile-dysfunction.
[8] Chan SW. Panax ginseng, Rhodiola rosea and Schisandra chinensis. Int J Food Sci Nutr. 2012 Mar;63 Suppl 1:75-81. doi: 10.3109/09637486.2011.627840.
[9] Freeman, D. Natural Remedies for Erectile Dysfunction. Accessed 21 April 2015 online at http://www.webmd.com/erectile-dysfunction/features/natural-remedies-for-erectile-dysfunction.
[10] Feldman HA, Goldstein I, et al. Impotence and its medical and psychosocial correlates: results of the Massachusetts Male Aging Study. J Urol. 1994 Jan;151(1):54-61.
[11] Freeman, D. Natural Remedies for Erectile

Dysfunction. Accessed 21 April 2015 online at
http://www.webmd.com/erectile-
dysfunction/features/natural-remedies-for-erectile-
dysfunction.

[12] Chen J, Wollman Y, et al. Effect of oral administration
of high-dose nitric oxide donor L-arginine in men with
organic erectile dysfunction: results of a double-blind,
randomized, placebo-controlled study. BJU Int. 1999
Feb;83(3):269-73.

[13] Aoki H, Nagao J, et al. Clinical assessment of a
supplement of Pycnogenol® and L-arginine in Japanese
patients with mild to moderate erectile dysfunction.
Phytother Res. 2012 Feb;26(2):204-7. doi:
10.1002/ptr.3462.

[14] Stanislavov R, Rohdewald P. Sperm quality in men is
improved by supplementation with a combination of L-
arginine, L-citrullin, roburins and Pycnogenol®. Minerva
Urol Nefrol. 2014 Dec;66(4):217-23.

[15] Kho HG, Sweep CG, et al. The use of acupuncture in
the treatment of erectile dysfunction. Int J Impot Res.
1999 Feb;11(1):41-6.

[16] Engelhardt PF, Daha LK, et al. Acupuncture in the
treatment of psychogenic erectile dysfunction: first
results of a prospective randomized placebo-controlled
study. Int J Impot Res. 2003 Oct;15(5):343-6.

[17] Suzuki E, Nishimatsu H, et al. Chronic kidney disease
and erectile dysfunction. World J Nephrol. 2014 Nov
6;3(4):220-9. doi: 10.5527/wjn.v3.i4.220.

[18] Forest CP, Padma-Nathan H, Liker HR. Efficacy and
safety of pomegranate juice on improvement of erectile
dysfunction in male patients with mild to moderate
erectile dysfunction: a randomized, placebo-controlled,
double-blind, crossover study. Int J Impot Res. 2007
Nov-Dec;19(6):564-7.

[19] Shindel AW1, Xin ZC, et al. Erectogenic and
neurotrophic effects of icariin, a purified extract of horny
goat weed (Epimedium spp.) in vitro and in vivo. J Sex
Med. 2010 Apr;7(4 Pt 1):1518-28. doi: 10.1111/j.1743-
6109.2009.01699.x.

[20] Cohen AJ, Bartlik B, et al. Ginkgo biloba for
antidepressant-induced sexual dysfunction. J Sex
Marital Ther. 1998 Apr-Jun;24(2):139-43.

[21] Leaf A, Albert CM, et al. Prevention of fatal arrhythmias in high-risk subjects by fish oil n-3 fatty acid intake. Circulation. 2005 Nov 1;112(18):2762-8.

[22] Shin ES, Garcia-Garcia HM, et al. Effect of statins on coronary bifurcation atherosclerosis: an intravascular ultrasound virtual histology study. Int J Cardiovasc Imaging. 2012 Oct;28(7):1643-52. doi: 10.1007/s10554-011-9989-9.

[23] Lee K, Ahn TH, et al. The effects of statin and niacin on plaque stability, plaque regression, inflammation and oxidative stress in patients with mild to moderate coronary artery stenosis. Korean Circ J. 2011 Nov;41(11):641-8. doi: 10.4070/kcj.2011.41.11.641.

[24] Wiehle RD, Fontenot GK, et al. Enclomiphene citrate stimulates testosterone production while preventing oligospermia: a randomized phase II clinical trial comparing topical testosterone. Fertil Steril. 2014 Sep;102(3):720-7. doi: 10.1016/j.fertnstert.2014.06.004.

[25] Lee K, Ahn TH, et al. The effects of statin and niacin on plaque stability, plaque regression, inflammation and oxidative stress in patients with mild to moderate coronary artery stenosis. Korean Circ J. 2011 Nov;41(11):641-8. doi: 10.4070/kcj.2011.41.11.641.

[26] Valentina VN, Marijan B, et al. Subclinical hypothyroidism and risk to carotid atherosclerosis. Arq Bras Endocrinol Metabol. 2011 Oct;55(7):475-80.

[27] Jiskra J, Límanová Z, et al. Autoimmune thyroid diseases in women with breast cancer and colorectal cancer. Physiol Res. 2004;53(6):693-702.

[28] Hellevik AI, Asvold BO, et al. Thyroid function and cancer risk: a prospective population study. Cancer Epidemiol Biomarkers Prev. 2009 Feb;18(2):570-4. doi: 10.1158/1055-9965.EPI-08-0911.

[29] Rajender S, Monica MG, et al. Thyroid, spermatogenesis, and male infertility. Front Biosci (Elite Ed). 2011 Jun 1;3:843-55.

[30] Von Radowitz, J. Daily sex keeps sperm healthy and improves chance of pregnancy. Accessed on 23 April 2015 online at http://www.independent.co.uk/life-style/health-and-families/health-news/daily-sex-keeps-sperm-healthy-and-improves-chance-of-pregnancy-1726197.html.